better nutrition *magazine presents*

OSTEOARTHRITIS

EFFECTIVELY ALLEVIATE PAIN

DOCTOR RECOMMENDED
Treatment Plan

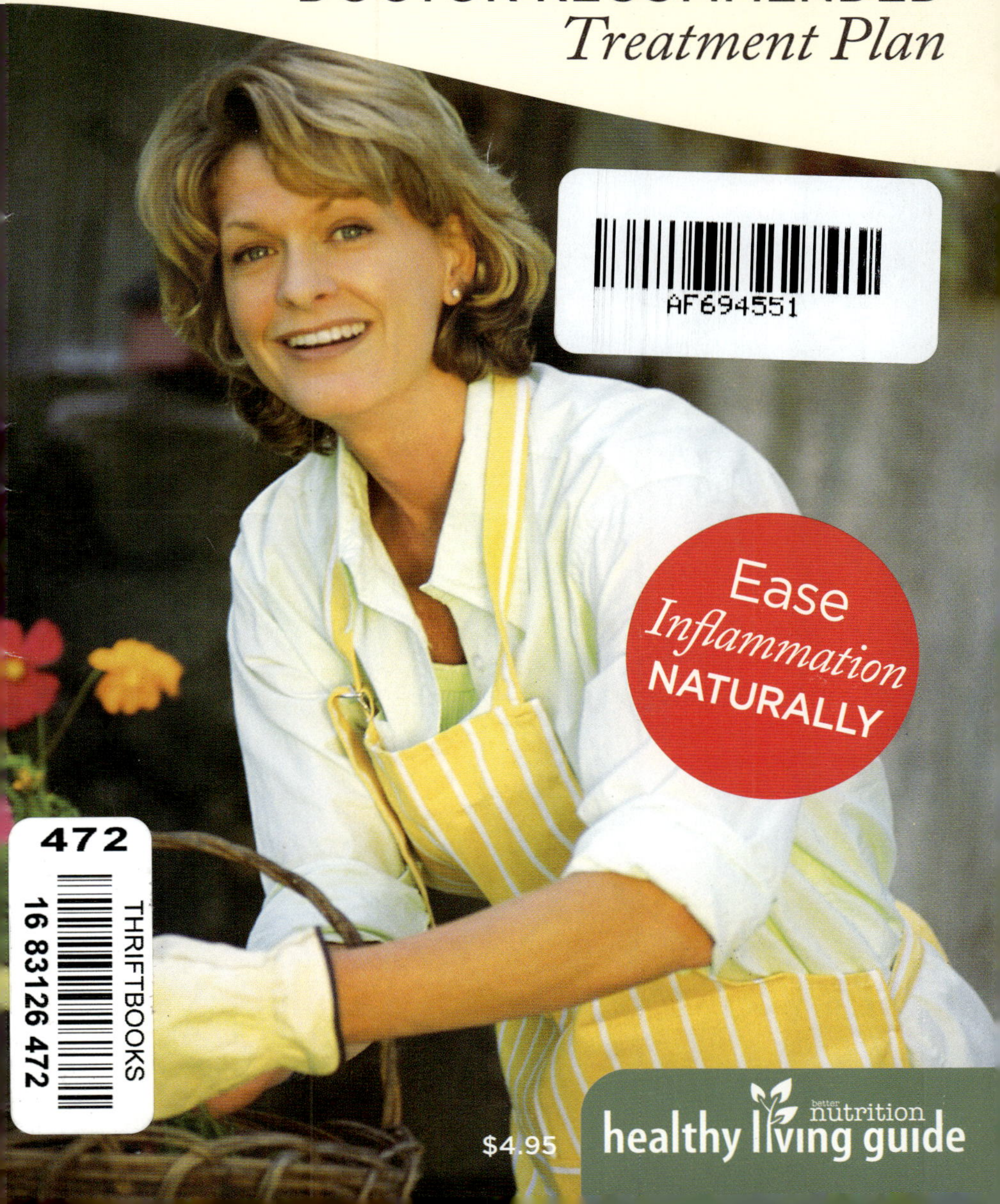

Ease *Inflammation* NATURALLY

$4.95

better nutrition healthy living guide

better nutrition *magazine* presents

OSTEOARTHRITIS

by LISE ALSCHULER, ND

better nutrition healthy living guide

Published by:
Active Interest Media, Inc.
300 N. Continental Blvd., Suite 650
El Segundo, CA 90245

This booklet is part of the *Better Nutrition Healthy Living Guide* series. For more information, visit www.betternutrition.com. Better Nutrition magazine is available at fine natural health stores throughout the United States. Design by Aline Design: Bellingham, Wash.

OSTEOARTHRITIS

CONTENTS

better nutrition
healthy living guide

Introduction

What is Osteoarthritis

Oh, those creaking joints, stiff back and sore knees—what a way to start the morning. Sadly, that is the way millions of Americans begin every day. Osteoarthritis, characterized mainly by joint pain and stiffness, is an uncomfortable and ominous accompaniment of adulthood for many. In fact, according to the National Institute of Arthritis and Musculoskeletal and Skin Diseases (NIAMS), 27 million Americans over the age of 25 are afflicted with osteoarthritis.

The incidence of osteoarthritis increases with age, and is second only to heart disease as a cause of work disability in men over age 50. Some joints may begin to show signs of osteoarthritis by the second or third decade of life, but these joints rarely cause symptoms at this age. By age 40, almost everyone has some osteoarthritic changes in their weight-bearing joints (hip and knee joints). And by age 75, osteoarthritis is present in virtually everyone.

Both men and women suffer from this potentially disabling disease. Before age 45, osteoarthritis is more common in men than women. But after age 45, it is more common in women. It is also more likely to occur in people who are overweight and in those who repeatedly engage in activities that stress particular joints. All things considered, when it comes to osteoarthritis, not many people are left out.

Despite its widespread prevalence, treatment for osteoarthritis is sorely lacking. The best that conventional medicine can do is manage the painful symptoms until joint replacement is the only option. While these measures can, and do, make a huge difference in the lives of those with osteoarthritis, people deserve to have better and different treatment options. The good news is that these options exist! Natural therapies, along with certain dietary and activity guidelines, can radically change one's experience with osteoarthritis. But, before we explore these treatments, let's learn a little more about osteoarthritis.

Osteoarthritis 101

Where the bones that make up our skeleton meet, a joint is made. Joints allow for the mobility of our bodies. Every movement that we make involves the action of a joint. Repetitive movements, especially in joints that bear weight, demand much from those joints. The way in which joints withstand this pressure is key to understanding osteoarthritis.

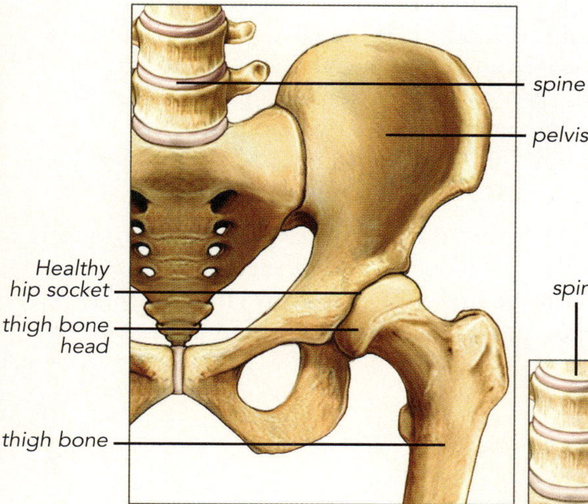

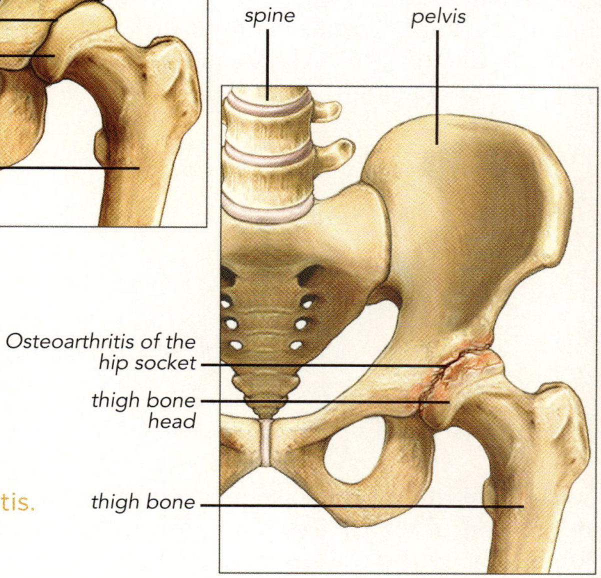

Hip Joints
Above, a healthy hip joint.
At right, osteoarthritis.

Joints are made up of the ends of two bones which are held together by tough strands of connective tissue known as fibrous ligaments. Joints are further supported by surrounding muscles and the tendons that attach muscle to bone. The joint space is contained within a tough capsule known as the joint capsule. Lining the inside of this joint capsule is the synovial membrane, or synovium. The synovium produces a small amount of thick fluid with an egg-like consistency called synovial fluid. The synovial fluid helps to nourish the cartilage and keep it slippery. Within the synovium, the ends of the bone are additionally cushioned with a spongy layer of cartilage covering each bone within the joint. The health and durability of cartilage is of key importance to the overall health of the joint.

One main component of cartilage is collagen. Collagen is a fibrous protein and is the main protein of all of our connective tissue, including cartilage. Collagen contributes great tensile strength to the cartilage. The other main component of joint cartilage is proteoglycans. Proteoglycans are proteins with glycosaminoglycan (GAG) sugar chains attached. Proteoglycans interlace with collagen to form a flexible mesh gel-like disc that absorbs the impacts on the joint, thereby cushioning the ends of the bones. We will learn more about proteoglycans later, as these molecules are critical components of protective cushion found in joints.

Chondrocytes are the only cells found in cartilage. These cells produce and maintain the collagen and proteoglycan cartilaginous matrix. The health of a joint depends upon the presence of healthy chondrocytes, as well as sufficient proteoglycan and collagen, to withstand the pressures placed upon that joint.

The destructive process of osteoarthritis is typically the result of wear-and-tear that develops over decades.

Osteoarthritis, also known as degenerative joint disease, results from destruction of the collagen and proteoglycan matrix of cartilage in the joints. One of the reasons that osteoarthritis is more common in older adults is that, as we age, the body's ability to repair and make new collagen and proteoglycans naturally decreases. Over time, the lack of sufficient collagen and proteoglycans destabilizes the joint and creates areas of pressure and friction between the bones that comprise the joint. In response to these pressure points, large bone spurs (calcified projections from the ends of the bones comprising the joint) develop. Subsequent movement of this joint causes the bone ends to grate on each other. This is particularly evident in a weight bearing joint, such as the hip or knee. This friction can cause significant pain.

The destructive process of osteoarthritis is typically the result of wear-and-tear that develops over decades. In some cases, joint trauma, congenital abnormalities of the joint or cartilage, or inflammatory diseases affecting the joint can set up the perfect conditions for the development of osteoarthritis at any age. Regardless of the origin, the process of joint destruction tends to be cumulative and progressive.

The Symptoms of Osteoarthritis

Sometimes osteoarthritic joints are without pain. More commonly, however, osteoarthritic joints definitely make their presence known! The first symptom of osteoarthritis is often a feeling of joint achiness after use. This is particularly true of weight bearing joints such as the back, hips and knees. Over time—usually years—this progresses to more constant joint pain and stiffness. Often, people will experience the most stiffness and pain upon waking in the morning and after remaining in one position for an extended period of time. Some arthritic joints will cause swelling and may produce an audible crunching feeling or sound upon movement of the joint.

Osteoarthritis can affect any joint and is most common in the hands (fingers), knees, hips and spine. Osteoarthritis of the hip is common in older adults and can cause pain in the groin, inner leg and buttocks. The pain of osteoarthritis in the hips can severely limit daily activities such as walking. Osteoarthritis of the spine can create pressure on the nerves that exit the spinal column in the vertebral joint spaces of the spine. This pressure inflames the exciting nerve and may result in numbness, tingling or pain in the arms or legs. Some osteoarthritic joints form bony nodules. Heberden's nodes can develop in ostearthritic joints of the fingers – the last joint in the finger. Bouchard's nodes can develop in the knuckle joints of the hands. These bony growths can be painful initially. But, while the pain subsides, the nodes deform the joint and limit its mobility.

Common Symptoms of Osteoarthritis

- Early morning joint stiffness
- Joint ache after use
- Constant joint pain and stiffness
- Joint swelling
- Bony nodules
- Audible crunching sound upon movement

Osteoarthritis can be confused with another type of arthritis called rheumatoid arthritis. Yet, while osteoarthritis is caused by wear-and-tear on joints, rheumatoid arthritis is an autoimmune disease in which the body's immune system produces antibodies that attack the connective tissue of certain joints. Rheumatoid arthritis is a serious systemic illness that requires medical management and which benefits from therapies that are different from those that benefit osteoarthritis.

Diagnosis

A visit to a physician with a complaint of joint pain or stiffness will inevitably involve a work-up for osteoarthritis. Osteoarthritis is initially diagnosed based on symptoms, and the diagnosis is then confirmed with radiographic studies (x-rays) of the afflicted joint(s). If x-rays do not confirm the diagnosis, the physician may order an MRI (Magnetic Resonance Imaging) in order to discover more subtle arthritic joint changes. Once diagnosed, typical medical management includes strategies to ease pain, improve joint function and reduce joint stress. Unfortunately, the treatment of osteoarthritis doesn't usually begin until it has already been well established in the body. This is unfortunate because there are certain medical conditions that increase the risk of developing osteoarthritis. People with these conditions would be well advised to support joint health before arthritis begins.

Osteoarthritis	Rheumatoid Arthritis
Affects women and men.	Affects 3 women to every 1 man.
Incidence increases with age, especially after the age of 40.	Occurs at any age, most commonly between the ages of 20 and 60.
Most common in weight bearing joints.	Most common in smaller joints (hands, wrist, feet).
Morning stiffness usually lasts less than 15 minutes.	Morning stiffness and stiffness after rest usually lasts longer than 15 minutes.
May only involve one joint (i.e. one hip or one knee).	Affects joints on both sides of the body (i.e. both hands and/or both feet).
Joints may appear normal.	Joints are red and swollen.
No systemic symptoms.	Systemic symptoms such as fatigue and fever.
No changes in blood tests.	Blood tests are positive for autoantibodies.

Causes

While osteoarthritis is generally the result of wear-and-tear on the affected joint, there are conditions that predispose the joint to this damage. Certainly, excess body weight adds to this wear-and-tear. With the rising rates of obesity in this country, more people than ever before will be affected with osteoarthritis.

Hormones like estrogen may also initiate or accelerate osteoarthritis. While estrogen is an important hormone in both women and men, excessive estrogen exposure should be minimized. Many of the synthetic compounds in our daily environment are estrogenic, so the overall estrogen influence in our bodies today is significantly stronger than in decades past.

Diabetics have a greater incidence of osteoarthritis, which may be the result of decreased insulin. Insulin plays a role in healthy joints because it stimulates chondrocytes to produce proteoglycans. Altered liver function, which can be the result of toxin-induced damage, malnutrition, infection or excessive fatty deposits, can also result in decreased production of cartilage repair hormones such as somatomedin. While osteoarthritis may not be entirely avoidable, addressing some of the conditions which can predispose someone to osteoarthritis is an important part of a holistic treatment plan. Unfortunately, conventional treatment of osteoarthritis typically focuses on simply controlling the symptoms.

Common Causes of Osteoarthritis

- Chronic wear and tear
- Aging (decreased cartilage production and repair)
- Joint trauma
- Congenital abnormalities
- Inflammatory diseases
- Obesity
- Diabetes
- Liver disease

Chapter One
Conventional Treatment

People seeking medical help for osteoarthritis are usually experiencing pain—thus the mainstay of conventional treatment is pain control. Conventional medicine does not speak to issues of cartilage preservation or repair, and does not address the underlying causes of osteoarthritis. Most conventional practitioners will recommend either aspirin or another non-steroidal anti-inflammatory drug (NSAID). NSAIDs decrease inflammation and pain by inhibiting the body's production of prostaglandins. Prostaglandins are natural chemicals which create inflammation and pain.

Aspirin, at fairly high doses (2,000 to 4,000 mg per day) can effectively reduce the pain of osteoarthritis. Many individuals can manage their pain for years with aspirin. However, aspirin—particularly at the dosage required for effective pain control—has significant side effects. The most common, and most dangerous, side effect is ulceration of the digestive tract. This occurs because prostaglandins are also important in maintaining a healthy and protected stomach lining. By disrupting the production of prostaglandins in the stomach, aspirin can cause ulcers and bleeding. Aspirin can also cause ringing in the ears (tinnitus).

Acetaminophen (Tylenol) is an analgesic drug that is also recommended for pain control. While this drug can effectively relieve pain, there are risks with long-term use. Acetaminophen can cause liver damage, increase the risk of certain heart problems, damage the digestive tract and cause rashes.

A commonly employed drug therapy for osteoarthritis includes non-aspirin NSAIDs such as ibuprofen (Motrin), indomethacin (Indocin) or naproxen (Naprosyn). These drugs can also effectively relieve the pain of osteoarthritis. Unfortunately, these drugs have side effects like dizziness, digestive bleeding and kidney damage. Additionally, NSAIDs inhibit the body's production of proteoglycans. This means that while the short-term effect of NSAIDs might be desired pain relief, the long-term effects include accelerated cartilage degeneration and the worsening of osteoarthritis!

Another type of pain medication that reduces the pain of osteoarthritis are COX-2 inhibitors. COX-2 inhibiting drugs like Celebrex were once

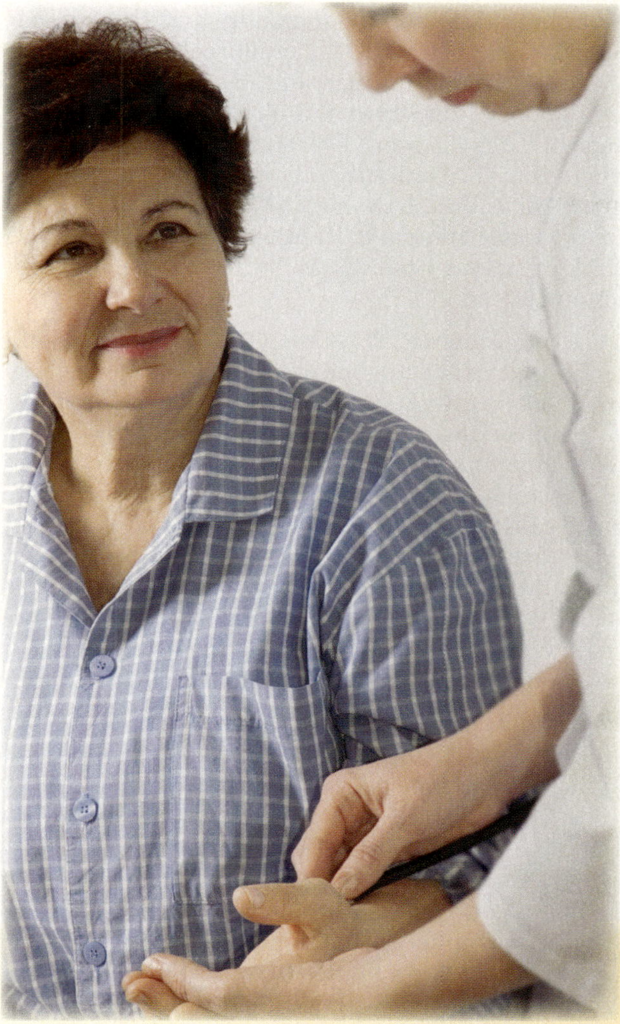

Conventional Osteoarthritis Treatments

- Aspirin
- NSAID
- Acetaminophen
- COX-2 inhibitor
- Corticosteroid injection
- Surgical joint replacement

thought to be a miracle anti-inflammatory and pain relieving medication because, unlike NSAIDs, COX-2 inhibitors do not inhibit the COX-1 enzyme. COX-1 is present throughout the body. It produces prostaglandins that mediate inflammation and increase the production of mucus. In the stomach, COX-1 is protective. So by leaving COX-1 activity intact, it was thought that COX-2 inhibitors would not cause ulceration of the digestive tract. But studies show that COX-2 inhibitors do increase the risk of digestive tract ulceration and bleeding. Of even greater concern is the increased risk of serious heart disease from COX-2 inhibitors, including heart attack and stroke.

If aspirin, acetaminophen, NSAIDs, COX-2 inhibitors or other prescription pain-relieving medications are unsuccessful at controlling the pain of osteoarthritis, other conventional strategies are employed. These include corticosteroid injections, which are usually given three to four times per year to relieve inflammatory flare-ups associated with osteoarthritis. Corticosteroid injections provide rapid pain relief, but also carry risk. These injections can cause tendons (the connective tissue that attaches muscle to bone) to weaken and even rupture. They can also introduce bacteria into the joint and aggravate inflammation. Corticosteroid injections also cannot be used too frequently or used long term since overuse can cause thinning of the skin, easy bruising, weight gain, puffiness of the face, elevation of blood pressure, cataract formation and osteoporosis.

The most definitive conventional treatment for osteoarthritis is surgery. There are several types of surgery used for severely damaged osteoarthritic joints, and these options are typically recommended as a way to improve joint function and to lessen pain. Surgery may remove loose pieces of bone and cartilage that are causing joint pain and instability. It can also be done to reposition the bones to stabilize the joint and to smooth the surfaces of the bones comprising the joint. If the joint is beyond repair and severely arthritic or painful, it can be surgically replaced with a prosthetic joint. There are various types of prostheses and surgical methods used to do these joint replacements. Most joint replacements last 10 to 15 years. Surgery can provide significant improvements to the quality of someone's life who has severe osteoarthritis. Nonetheless, the expense of surgery, along with the risk inherent with any surgery, makes this conventional option a treatment of last resort.

Chapter Two
Natural Options

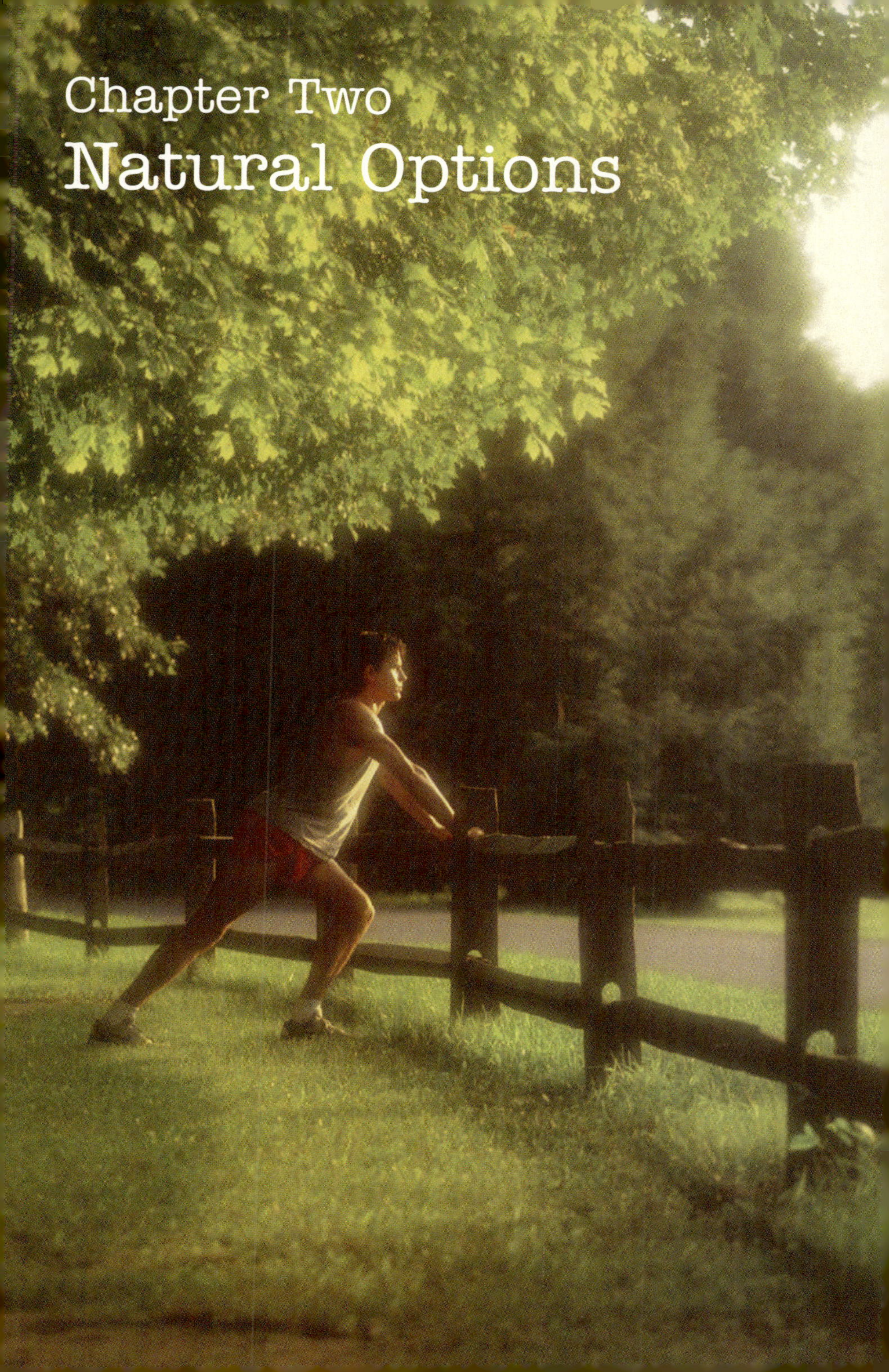

Conventional treatment of osteoarthritis leaves much to be desired. The price of pain relief from these mainstream treatments is a combination of side effects and continued joint deterioration. Fortunately, there are effective natural therapies that not only reduce pain, they actually improve the health of osteoarthritic joints. The goal of these natural therapies is to reduce inflammation, stimulate cartilage repair, reduce pain and increase the overall integrity of the joint.

Glucosamine Sulfate

Natural treatment of osteoarthritis gained significant attention with the introduction of glucosamine sulfate in the 1980's. Glucosamine is a small molecule that stimulates the production of glycosaminoglycans (GAGs), the main proteoglycan in joint cartilage. Proteoglycans cushion the joint and their presence is critical to pain-free, fluid movement. Glucosamine also helps stabilize the other component of cartilage, namely the fibrous collagen.

Glucosamine is essential to both the cushioning gel and the collagen scaffolding of cartilage. It attenuates—and may even reverse—the hallmark cartilage destruction of osteoarthritic joints. Glucosamine has been the subject of several clinical trials in people with the disease. In these trials, it appreciably improves pain and movement of osteoarthritic joints over a placebo. There appear to be no side effects and long-term use is associated with even greater benefit. Typically, 500 mg of glucosamine is taken three times daily.

It's important to note, however, that glucosamine is not effective for everyone who uses it. Fortunately, since the introduction of glucosamine, several new natural therapies have been introduced that promise to take the natural management of osteoarthritis to an entirely different level.

Herbal Management of Osteoarthritis

As technology continues to shrink our world, the globalization of many industries has enriched and expanded the inventory of things available to consumers. One industry which has clearly benefitted from this globalization is the botanical industry. Herbs that were once used exclusively in remote regions of the world are now the subject of scientific studies around the globe. It is also now possible to combine herbal extracts from diverse parts of the world into powerful synergistic formulas. As a result, people with diseases like osteoarthritis can benefit in a way that was not possible decades ago.

One such herbal combination that promises help to people with osteoarthritis combines herbs from India, the Middle East and Africa.

These herbs each have a robust tradition of use for joint discomfort in their respective places of origin. Each herb has also been studied using modern scientific methods to confirm their benefits. The herbs are *Boswellia serrate* (frankincense), *Curcuma longa* (turmeric), *Harpagophytum procumbens* (Devil's claw) and *Emblica officinalis* (Indian gooseberry or amla).

Synergism between herbal extracts means that the combined benefits are far greater than those from each individual herbal component. This same principle is true for the herbs themselves.

Concentrated extracts of these herbs combine to make a potent anti-arthritic formula. Although much of the research on herbal therapies is done on individual herbs, herbalists and naturopathic physicians often combine more than one herb to treat a certain indication. The overlapping effects of each herb are more than additive they are synergistic. Synergism between herbal extracts means that the combined benefits are far greater than those from each individual herbal component. This same principle is true for the herbs themselves and is one reason why herbal therapy is so compelling.

Even though these extracts concentrate certain compounds naturally found in the plant, the whole plant is retained in the final extraction. While we may not know about the medicinal value of each compound in a plant, herbal medicine understands that there likely is value in all parts of the plant and that combined effect is a synergistic one. This concept is a hallmark of herbal medicine and may help to explain why herbal medicines, while apparently much less concentrated than their drug counterparts, are so successful. The following combination of herbal extracts is one example of a powerful and synergistic plant-based medicine.

Boswellia (*Boswellia serrata*) extract standardized to contain greater than 70 percent boswellic acid with acetyl-11-keto-beta-boswellic acid (AKBA) greater than 10 percent.

Curcumin (*Curcuma longa*) CRX 791 rhizome extract with curcuminoid complex (curcumin, demethoxycurcumin and bisdemethoxycurcumin).

Devil's claw (*Harpagophytum procumbens*) extract standardized to contain greater than 20 percent harpagosides (by HPLC).

Indian Gooseberry (*Emblica officinalis*) extract standardized to contain greater than 30 percent total polyphenols content with emblicanins greater than 20 percent.

Recommended dosage: 1,050 mg of this combination daily.

In order to understand the combined effect that these herbs create, let's look at each herb in detail.

Boswellia serrata (Frankincense)

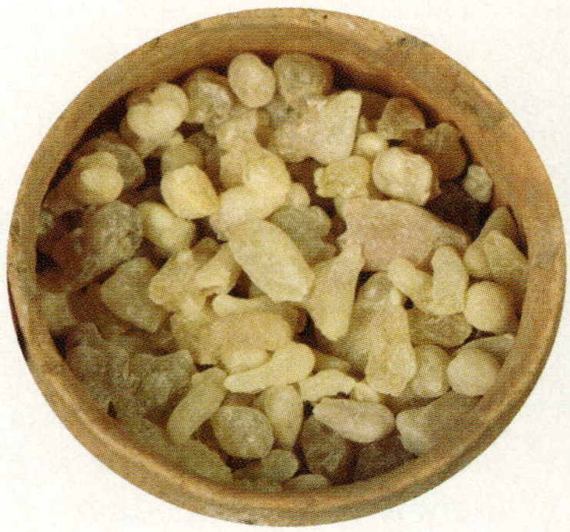

Frankincense: The boswellia tree exudes a gum resin.

Boswellia is a botanical which has proven effective in the management of arthritis. The boswellia tree grows in the Middle East and India. Incisions made in the trunk of this tree exude a gum resin that is collected after allowing it to harden. The gum oleoresin consists of essential oils and gum, as well as terpenoids that contain boswellic acids. Boswellic acids, the biologically active ingredients of the gum resin, are specific, non-competitive inhibitors of 5-lipoxygenase—the key enzyme that converts arachidonic acid into leukotrienes. Arachidonic acid, sometimes referred to as a pro-inflammatory fat, is a polyunsaturated fat found primarily in red meat, egg yolk and organ meat. Arachidonic acid is used to synthesize important regulatory molecules such as prostaglandins (chemical messengers), thromboxanes (involved in platelet aggregation) and leukotrienes. Leukotrienes are bioactive lipids that play a central role in sustaining inflammation. An overabundance of leukotrienes will increase inflammation in the body. Boswellic acids inhibit 5-lipoxygenase and, in so doing, decrease inflammation.

The anti-inflammatory actions of boswellia are so pronounced that this herb is considered to be primarily an anti-inflammatory herb. As a result, it is useful for treating arthritis, asthma, bronchitis, laryngitis and inflammatory skin conditions. Unlike conventional anti-inflammatory drugs, the long-term use of boswellia does not lead to irritation or ulceration of the stomach. This is because boswellia does not inhibit COX-1 or COX-2 enzymes.

There are many boswellic acids in boswellia extract, but these acids don't all act alike. In fact, one of the acids—ß-boswellic acid—found in most commercial extracts of boswellia may actually activate arachidonic acid and 5-lipoxygenase—the very opposite of what is intended. In contrast, acetyl boswellic acids (namely acetyl-11-keto-ß-Boswellic acid or AKBA) have the most potent 5-lipoxygenase inhibitory—and therefore anti-inflammatory—action. Most commercial boswellia products are standardized to contain either 65 percent or 75 to 85 percent boswellic acids. However, there are six different boswellic acids present in these extracts, with the pro-inflammatory ß-boswellic acid being the major one. What's more, these extracts only contain one to three percent of the anti-inflammatory AKBA. The most potent anti-inflammatory boswellia products should be standardized to contain at least 70 percent boswellic acids with greater than 10 percent AKBA and no ß-boswellic acid. While this may seem confusing, it is important to know how to evaluate a good product in order to obtain the benefits of this important botanical extract.

The anti-inflammatory action of boswellic acids treat osteoarthritis by helping to control pain and by reducing the inflammatory component of cartilage destruction. In addition, boswellic acids support proteoglycan synthesis (which provide cushion to the joint), and improve blood supply to the joint. A dietary supplement containing boswellia was studied and found to produce a significant drop in the severity of pain and disability in the patients with osteoarthritis. This study, which was placebo-controlled, involved 42 patients who were evaluated over a period of eight months. An x-ray assessment of the arthritic joints did not show any significant changes, even though the symptoms improved. The trial was not long enough to demonstrate any increases in cartilage, but it does indicate that boswellia is effective in reducing pain. The dosage range for boswellia extracts that are standardized to at least 70 percent boswellic acids and no less than 10 percent AKBA is from 400 to 800 mg three times daily.

Curcuma longa (Turmeric)

Turmeric is a culinary spice and a critical ingredient of the curries of India, Indonesia and China where this plant grows. Turmeric root is usually boiled, cleaned and dried, yielding a yellow powder. One important component of turmeric is curcumin, a complex of several curcuminoids including curcumin (diferuloylmethane), demethoxycurcumin and disdemethoxycurcumin. Curcuminoids possess significant antioxidant, lipid lowering, anti-cancer and anti-inflammatory effects. In addition, volatile oils found in turmeric root are anti-inflammatory. The anti-inflammatory effects of curcumin are what make this plant so effective in the treatment of osteoarthritis.

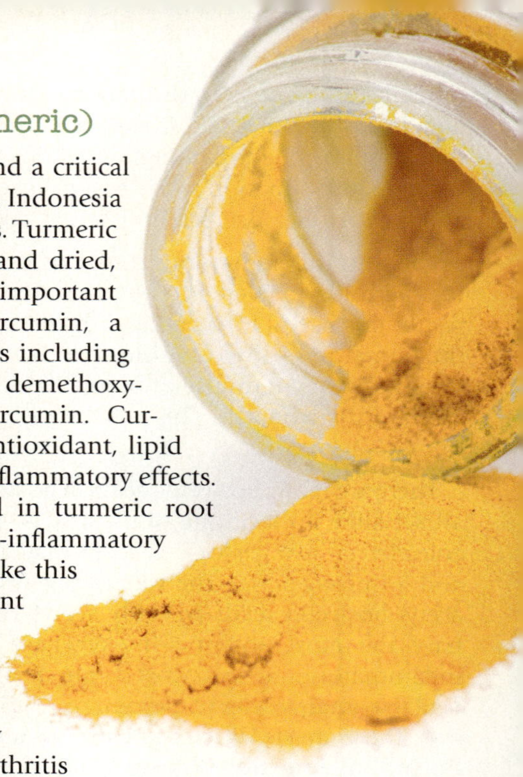

Turmeric powder

While osteoarthritis is not considered an inflammatory disease, inflammation does play an important role. As osteoarthritis progresses, tissue injury results from the eroding cartilage that normally cushions the joint. This injury triggers the release of inflammatory chemicals that further erode the cartilage, cause fluid to leak into the tissues of the joint and induce joint swelling. This swelling compresses nerve endings and causes pain. While inflammation is not the original cause of osteoarthritis, it does contribute to the diseases' progression and causes joint pain.

This brings us back to turmeric. Turmeric extract, concentrated to curcumin and its curcuminoids, is a potent anti-inflammatory agent. When administered orally, curcumin inhibits the biosynthesis of inflammatory prostaglandins and leukotrienes from arachidonic acid. It also inhibits the synthesis, release and activity of many other inflammatory mediators secreted by immune cells during a normal inflammatory response. Animal studies have demonstrated that curcumin is more effective than cortisone in relieving acute inflammation and in reducing inflammatory swelling. Curcumin is also effective (although less so than cortisone) in relieving chronic inflammation. In clinical trials, curcumin (1,200 mg per day) is as effective as the powerful arthritis drug phenylbutazone (300 mg per day) in relieving the symptoms of rheumatoid arthritis (morning stiffness, joint swelling) without the side effects of the drug. Curcumin (400 mg) is also equivalent to ibuprofen (400 mg) for reducing post-operative inflammation, although curcumin does not possess the side effects of ibuprofen.

One of the challenges with turmeric is the poor bioavailability of the curcuminoids. Although, orally dosed curcumin is without toxicity at large doses—even up to 12,000 mg in a single dose—excessively large amounts are required to result in any appreciable quantities in the blood and body tissues. These doses make typical turmeric extracts an unrealistic therapy. An oral dose of 8,000 mg of curcumin extract standardized to 95 percent curcuminoids, which represents the majority of curcumin commercially available products, is required to produce even low levels of curcumin in the blood. One would have to take about 16 capsules of this extract every day to achieve this dose. In an effort to reduce the dose, some extracts combine piperine (extracted from black pepper) with curcuminoids in order to increase the absorption of the curcuminoids. While this does result in more bioavailability, the difference is not great enough to substantially reduce the dosing requirements of these products. Fortunately, a new methodology for preparing turmeric extracts has finally made this herb a viable therapy.

Thanks to this breakthrough, a curcumin extract (known as BCM-95 or also CRX 791) has been introduced that utilizes micronized curcumin rhizome extract, phospholipids and turmeric essential oils to create increased bioavailability of the curcuminoids. Preliminary studies indicate that CRX 791 results in up to eight times more bioavailability than curcumin 95 percent extract and seven times more bioavailability than curcumin combined with piperine. Furthermore, CRX 791 remains in the blood for more than eight hours as opposed to the four to five hours seen with curcumin 95 percent extract. A toxicology study has demonstrated that this new extract is safe and without adverse toxicity. Bottom line: taking 600 mg of CRX 791 curcumin extract has the approximate bioequivalence of using 4,000 mg of curcumin 95 percent extract or 85,000 mg of dried turmeric root. What's more, 600 mg of CRX 791 fits into one capsule, making curcumin a realistic therapy to effectively treat the pain and inflammation of osteoarthritis.

Harpagophytum procumbens (Devil's claw)

Devil's claw is native to the arid southwestern regions of Africa. The plant derives its name from its fruit, which looks like a large hooked claw. The root of the plant has been used medicinally by African natives for centuries to treat rheumatic and gastrointestinal complaints. Because of Devil's claw's potent anti-inflammatory properties, it is now used worldwide for treating arthritis. The anti-inflammatory activity of Devil's claw is so powerful that its efficacy has been compared with cortisone.

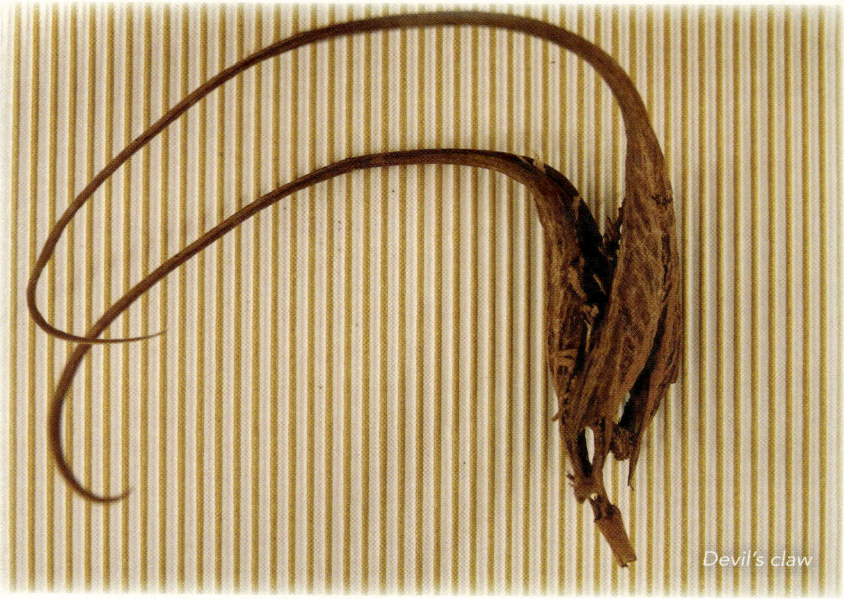

Devil's claw

Devil's claw also possesses notable pain relieving effects. It also dilates blood vessels, thus increasing circulation of nutrient-rich blood to, and waste-laden blood away from, the joints. This combination of anti-inflammatory, analgesic and vasodilatory actions results in decreased joint swelling and pain.

The substances responsible for the anti-arthritis actions of Devil's claw are iridoids, especially harpagoside. These iridoids represent 0.1 to 3.0 percent of the dried root. Recent advances in technology have allowed for the production of an extract with 20 percent (by HPLC) harpagosides, which effectively maximizes the plant's anti-arthritis actions. Because this herbal extract inhibits the COX-2 enzyme, it decreases the body's production of inflammatory prostaglandins, notably in the joints. This extract also stimulates chondrocytes to produce glycosaminoglycans (GAGs)—the key proteoglycans that cushion the joint. Finally, this extract stimulates the synthesis of hyaluronic acid by chondrocytes. Hyaluronic acid is part of the matrix surrounding cells and its presence reduces inflammatory tissue damage. This concentrated extract of Devil's claw exerts all of the actions required to slow down, and perhaps even reverse, the progression of osteoarthritic joint degeneration. This plant has already been proven to reduce the symptoms associated with osteoarthritis.

Devil's claw has been the subject of several human studies on people with arthritis. A review of all studies conducted on Devil's claw between 1966 and 2006 assessed the safety and efficacy of this extract and concluded that

Devil's claw has no acute toxicity and only mild adverse effects like diarrhea and flatulence. The efficacy of Devil's claw was more difficult to conclude given the wide variety of extracts and dosages used. Nonetheless, there was indication of superior pain relief from the use of Devil's claw extracts.

One study included 222 adults with mild to moderate joint disease. The subjects were given 960 mg of Devil's claw extract for eight weeks. Over the course of the study, more than half of the patients rated the Devil's claw extract as "excellent" and scores for pain, daily function and stiffness improved significantly. There were no serious adverse reactions reported by any of the participants. Several randomized, placebo-controlled clinical trials on patients with osteoarthritis of the knee, hip or back also demonstrated significant pain relief over eight to 16 weeks of use.

It is recommended that those suffering from osteoarthritis obtain two to five grams of the root powder (yielding an average of 30 mg harpagoside) and take it daily. It typically takes at least two months before pain reduction is experienced. The daily dose of the potent extract, which is standardized to contain 20 percent (by HPLC) harpagosides, is 200 mg in order to provide 40 mg harpagosides.

Emblica officinalis (Indian Gooseberry)

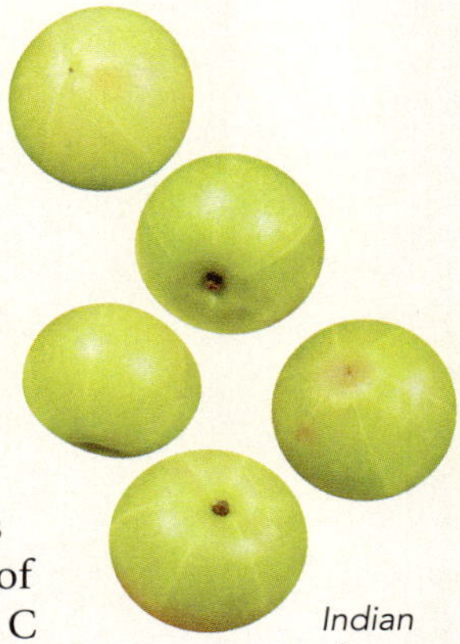

Indian gooseberry

Indian Gooseberry, also known as amla, is another important component in the comprehensive treatment of osteoarthritis. Indian gooseberry is native to India and its sour fruit has traditionally been used to treat liver disorders, intestinal diseases and joint diseases. Modern research has identified several unique compounds and characteristics of this plant. Indian gooseberry is one of the richest sources of vitamin C known, containing 30 times more vitamin C as oranges. Vitamin C (ascorbic acid) is a critical nutrient for those afflicted with osteoarthritis, since it is necessary for chondrocytes to make cartilage. In particular, vitamin C is needed for the production of the shock-absorbing proteoglycans in the joint. When animals with osteoarthritic joints are fed high doses of vitamin C, there is significantly less joint erosion and more stable proteoglycans.

In addition to the vitamin C found in Indian gooseberries, there are several other compounds in this fruit that lend it potent antioxidative and anti-inflammatory benefits. These compounds are polyphenols known as emblicanins. Emblicanins, particularly emblicanin-A and emblicanin-B, quench the free radicals that contribute to osteoarthritis.

Chronic tissue damage—including the damage found in osteoarthritic joints—is mediated, in part, by oxidative damage to the tissues that comprise the joint. Oxidative damage occurs when very reactive compounds known as free radicals react with normal cells, resulting in the damage, and often death, of those cells. They are produced in injured tissues as a part of the inflammatory healing response. Free radicals are an important part of acute inflammation because they stimulate immune activity and tissue repair. Nonetheless, there is such a thing as too much of a good thing where free radicals are concerned. As the healing progresses, the free radicals are normally quenched by antioxidant compounds—a necessary step to avoid unchecked and widespread tissue damage. Unfortunately, tissues that sustain repeated trauma, such as an osteoarthritic joint, will be exposed to free radicals day in and day out. The antioxidative capacity of the joint is used up. This long exposure to free radicals can cause serious oxidative damage to the joint. This is where antioxidants, such as vitamin C and emblicanins, come in.

Emblicans restore these antioxidants as they quench free radicals. The overall result is sustained antioxidant activity in the damaged joint.

Emblicanins are among the most potent plant-based antioxidants. Emblicanins, namely emblicanin-A and emblicanin-B, regenerate not only themselves, but vitamin C and the body's own antioxidants such as super oxide dismutase (SOD), catalase and glutathione. Emblicans restore these antioxidants as they, themselves, quench free radicals. The overall result is sustained antioxidant activity in the damaged joint. This would seem to be the perfect fit for a chronic oxidative state such as that found in osteoarthritis. In fact, in an animal study, those with arthritic joints experienced considerably less inflammation after being given an Indian gooseberry extract. The antioxidant actions of Indian gooseberry extract also increases collagen production. Collagen, a major component of cartilage, is produced by chrondrocytes. Under oxidative stress, chondrocytes are damaged and their ability to produce collagen is decreased.

The potent antioxidative properties of Indian gooseberry extract offers some protection to chondrocytes from oxidative damage, preserving their ability to produce collagen (and proteoglycans). The long-term chondroprotective activity of Indian gooseberry extract on human arthritis is comparable to that of glucosamine sulfate in terms of magnitude and potency. In contrast to glucosamine, Indian gooseberries induce a strong chondroprotective response in cartilage from patients with chronic osteoarthritis. Glucosamine exerts a chondroprotective response in some, but not all chronic osteoarthritis sufferers.

Indian gooseberry is most effective as a standardized extract. Most extracts are standardized to 1.0 to1.5 percent vitamin C and 30 to 45 percent polyphenols (tannins). These extracts are made from commercially grown and harvested dried fruits. While the drying process liberates the vitamin C, the dried fruit condenses the polyphenols, including the emblicanins. Unfortunately, condensed polyphenols are not bioavailable. As potent as vitamin C is, this plant derives a hefty portion of its antioxidant activity from the polyphenols, too. Extracts which utilize freshly juiced wild Indian gooseberries (higher in vitamin C than commercially grown hybrid crops) retain the polyphenols. The polyphenols are combined with vitamin C resulting in a very bioavailable and stable vitamin C-polyphenol complex. This extract is standardized to contain a minimum of 30 percent total polyphenols of which at least 20 percent is emblicanins. This potent extract is dosed between 500 mg and 1,000 mg daily.

These four herbs are wonderfully effective solutions to osteoarthritis. The combination of traditional medicine and modern extraction technology has yielded potent botanical medicines from them. Combining the most effective botanicals creates a superior pain-relieving, anti-inflammatory and cartilage-restoring medicine. As mentioned previously, the desired combination is:

- Boswellia (*Boswellia serrata*) extract standardized to contain greater than 70 percent boswellic acid with AKBA greater than 10 percent.
- Curcumin (*Curcuma longa*) CRX 791 rhizome extract with curcuminoids complex (curcumin, demethoxycurcumin and bisdemethoxycurcumin).
- Devil's claw (*Harpagophytum procumbens*) extract standardized to contain greater than 20 percent harpagosides (by HPLC).
- Indian Gooseberry (*Emblica officinalis*) extract standardized to contain greater than 30 percent total polyphenols content with emblicanins greater than 20 percent.

Recommended dosage: 1,050 mg of this combination daily.

Chapter Three

Adopt an Anti-Inflammatory Diet

Regardless of how potent herbal therapies and supplements are in the treatment of osteoarthritis, lifestyle habits are the true foundation for success. Diet and exercise are of utmost importance in the management of osteoarthritis. Learning how to use your diet and your activity as tools for healthier joints is both practical and empowering.

The primary basis for good health—and healthy joints—is a whole foods diet. A whole foods diet is mainly comprised of foods that are minimally processed. The diet should contain a colorful array of vegetables and fruit, plenty of whole grains, legumes, seeds and nuts, adequate water and high quality protein sources like soy, fish, poultry, antibiotic-free meat and eggs. A whole foods diet has minimal to no processed foods, refined grains, excessive fat or alcohol. This diet is also known as an anti-inflammatory diet.

A whole foods diet contains adequate vitamins, minerals, flavonoids and essential fatty acids for healthy joints. These nutrients provide direct antioxidant activity, and supply the required co-factors for essential enzyme activity and optimal tissue function. They also support healthy cell membranes. All of these actions reduce inflammation. A whole foods diet is also devoid of processed foods and excess sugar which damage tissue integrity and promote inflammatory pathways. The anti-inflammatory whole foods diet is an important foundation for those with osteoarthritis.

The virtues of a whole foods diet are many, including its impact on weight management. This is an important consideration for those with osteoarthritis since carrying excess weight adds pressure to weight-bearing joints—the very joints most likely to be affected with osteoarthritis. A number of studies have shown that obesity represents one of the most important risk factors for the disease. Excess weight is also a key predictor for the progression of osteoarthritis. The link between obesity and osteoarthritis is most evident for the weight bearing joints, namely the knee and hip. In fact, the connection is linear—the more weight a person gains, the greater their risk for osteoarthritis in their weight-bearing joints. Additionally, the longer someone is obese, the greater their risk for osteoarthritis development and progression. Almost one-third of all hip replacements are the result of obesity, and two-thirds of knee replacements are attributed to being overweight.

Interestingly, obesity also increases the risk of osteoarthritis of non-weight bearing joints such as the joints of the hand. This is thought to be due to the fact that obese individuals have different levels of certain hormones, such as leptin, secreted from their fat cells which may aggravate joint degeneration. Clearly, weight loss in obese individuals is of critical importance. Even a relatively modest weight reduction of five percent of body weight can result in a significant improvement in the symptoms of osteoarthritis. Of course, given that the relationship between weight and osteoarthritis is linear, the closer to ideal body weight that a person can be, the less likely he/she will be to develop or worsen osteoarthritis. A whole foods, anti-inflammatory diet also happens to be an excellent weight reduction diet. Adhering to this nutritious way of eating will convey significant joint health benefits (refer to the sidebar A Day in the Life of a Whole Foods Diet on page 26).

Anti-Arthritis Superfoods

Within the broad guidelines of eating a whole foods diet, certain foods deserve special emphasis for their unique roles in preserving healthy joints. Key foods to emphasize are berries, eggs, legumes, garlic, onions, cabbage, brussels sprouts and ginger. Berries are important sources of the plant pigments collectively referred to as flavonoids. Flavonoids have strong antioxidant and anti-inflammatory properties. The flavonoids in fruits like blueberries, raspberries, blackberries and strawberries, as well as cherries and grapes—consumed regularly over many years—will decrease oxidative inflammation throughout the body, joints included.

Also important are sulfur-containing foods such as eggs, legumes, garlic, onions, Brussels sprouts and cabbage. Sulfur is required to help cross-link the collagen fibers that form the structure of cartilage. A sulfur deficiency will impair the integrity of cartilage and will hasten the development of osteoarthritis.

Another important inclusion in the diet is ginger. Ginger root contains volatile oils, namely gingerols, which are potent anti-inflammatory agents. Daily consumption of ginger, even as little as a quarter-inch of the root can lessen the pain and swelling of osteoarthritis.

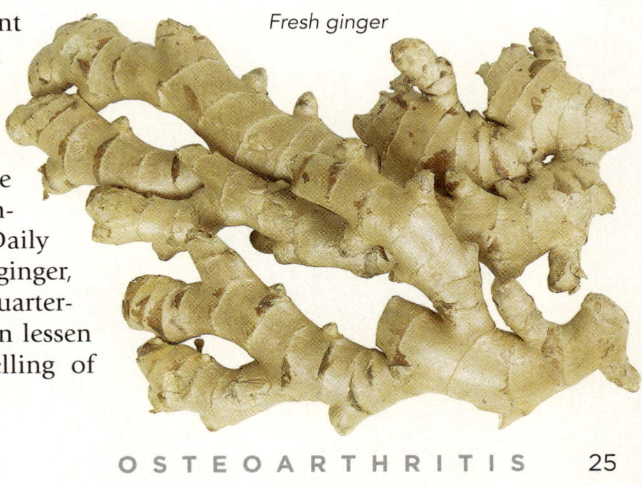

Fresh ginger

A Day in the Life of a Whole Foods Diet

Filling your plate with these anti-inflammatory foods may help tamp down the symptoms of osteoarthritis:

- **Plentiful fruits and vegetables:** At least six to eight daily servings of colorful vegetables and fruits. Opt for organic whenever possible. One serving = 1 cup raw vegetable or fruit = 1/2 cup cooked vegetable)
- **Whole grains:** At least one to two daily servings of brown rice, oats, whole wheat, etc.
- **Healthy fats:** One to two servings of avocado, olive oil, nuts, seeds and fatty fish. Oils should be minimally processed and should not be heated to high temperatures.
- **Legumes:** At least one to two daily servings of beans or peas.
- **Protein from eggs and lean meats:** One to two daily servings of eggs, chicken, pork and fish, organic if possible.
- **Water:** Eight cups daily.

This healthy weight, anti-inflammatory diet should minimize added sugar, alcohol, soft drinks, refined carbohydrates, fried foods, excessive red meat and smoked or processed meat. If poor digestion is an issue, oral digestive enzymes or pepsin hydrochloride may be helpful with meals.

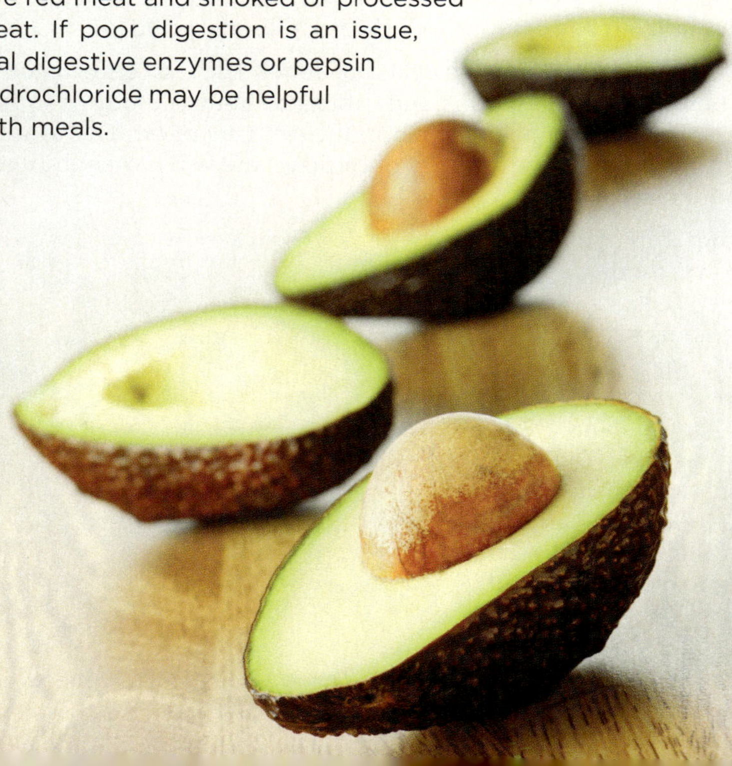

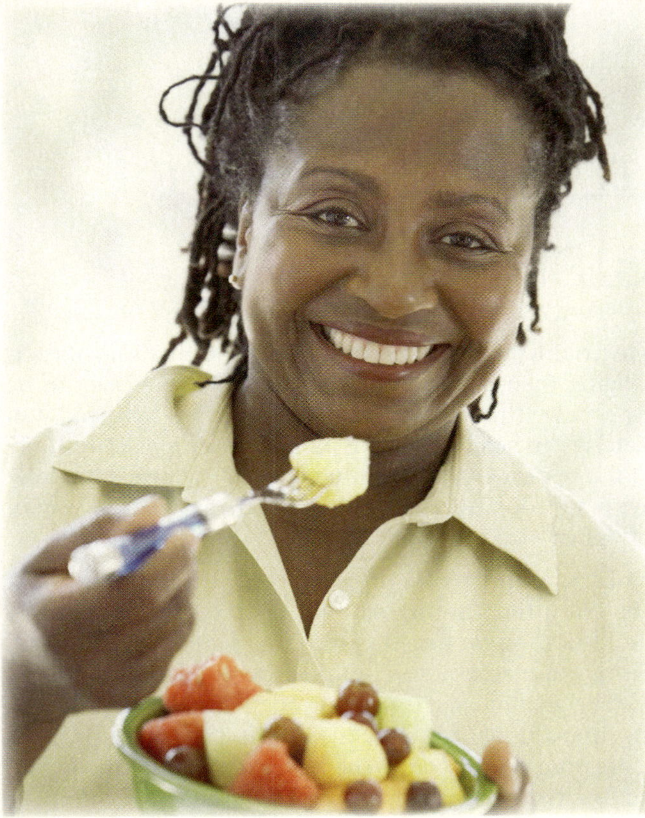

The flavonoids in fruits like blueberries, raspberries, blackberries and strawberries will decrease oxidative inflammation throughout the body, joints included.

Foods to Avoid

As important as beneficial foods are, the avoidance of joint-damaging food is also critical. One such food group to consider avoiding is the solanaceae (nightshade) family, which includes tomatoes, white potatoes, eggplant, peppers and tobacco. These foods contain a compound called solanine which, in some people, may inhibit collagen repair in damaged joints. Some people are more sensitive to this compound than others. A trial avoidance of all nightshade family foods for three to six months will help determine if this compound is worsening the discomfort of osteoarthritic joints.

Highly processed foods, such as refined grains, white sugar and alcohol, as well as the saturated fats in red meat and dairy, promote inflammation. These foods favor the production of inflammatory prostaglandins and leukotrienes, disrupt cell membrane homeostasis and influence the production of inflammatory hormones such as leptin and insulin. Inflammation facilitates joint degeneration. Eliminating these foods on a trial basis, for three to six months, may result in significant improvements in joint pain and mobility.

Chapter Four

The Importance of Exercise

People with osteoarthritis are often confused about the role of exercise in managing their disease. On the one hand, exercise can be painful—especially if the weight-bearing joints are involved. On the other hand, exercise can actually reduce pain and improve joint function, particularly if the correct exercise is done. Proper exercise, especially when combined with appropriate weight loss, can be a powerful way to improve the symptoms of osteoarthritis.

Proper exercise has a number of components. The most important aspect of exercise is that it be non-traumatic. Someone with osteoarthritis of the knee should not jog on paved roads. This same person would, however, benefit from water aerobics or an individually-designed weight resistance program. The goal of exercise is to strengthen the muscles, tendons and ligaments supporting the joint while minimizing pounding, jarring and excessive pressure on the joint. The best exercises are those that are low-impact and low-resistance such as bicycling, walking, swimming, rowing, isometrics and low-resistance strength training. High-impact exercises such as running, jumping and heavy weight training can aggravate osteoarthritic joints. Any exercise that causes noticeable or prolonged joint pain should be avoided. All exercise should be followed with stretching in order to encourage joint mobility.

Exercise is important for people with osteoarthritis. People who are poorly conditioned and who have weak supporting musculature suffer from more pain and joint dysfunction. Strong muscles support the joint and, in so doing, decrease joint wear-and-tear. Additionally, muscle contractions pump fluid into and out of joints. Cartilage has a limited blood supply and is dependent upon muscle movement for the influx of nutrients and the removal of waste. Nutrients are necessary for adequate cartilage production and repair. Wastes need to be removed in order to avoid oxidative damage and inflammation. Proper exercise supports healthy cartilage and enhances the structural integrity of the joint.

It is important for the joint to be well supported during exercise. Individuals with osteoarthritis of the hip or knee should obtain a postural and orthopedic evaluation. Any structural abnormalities putting strain on

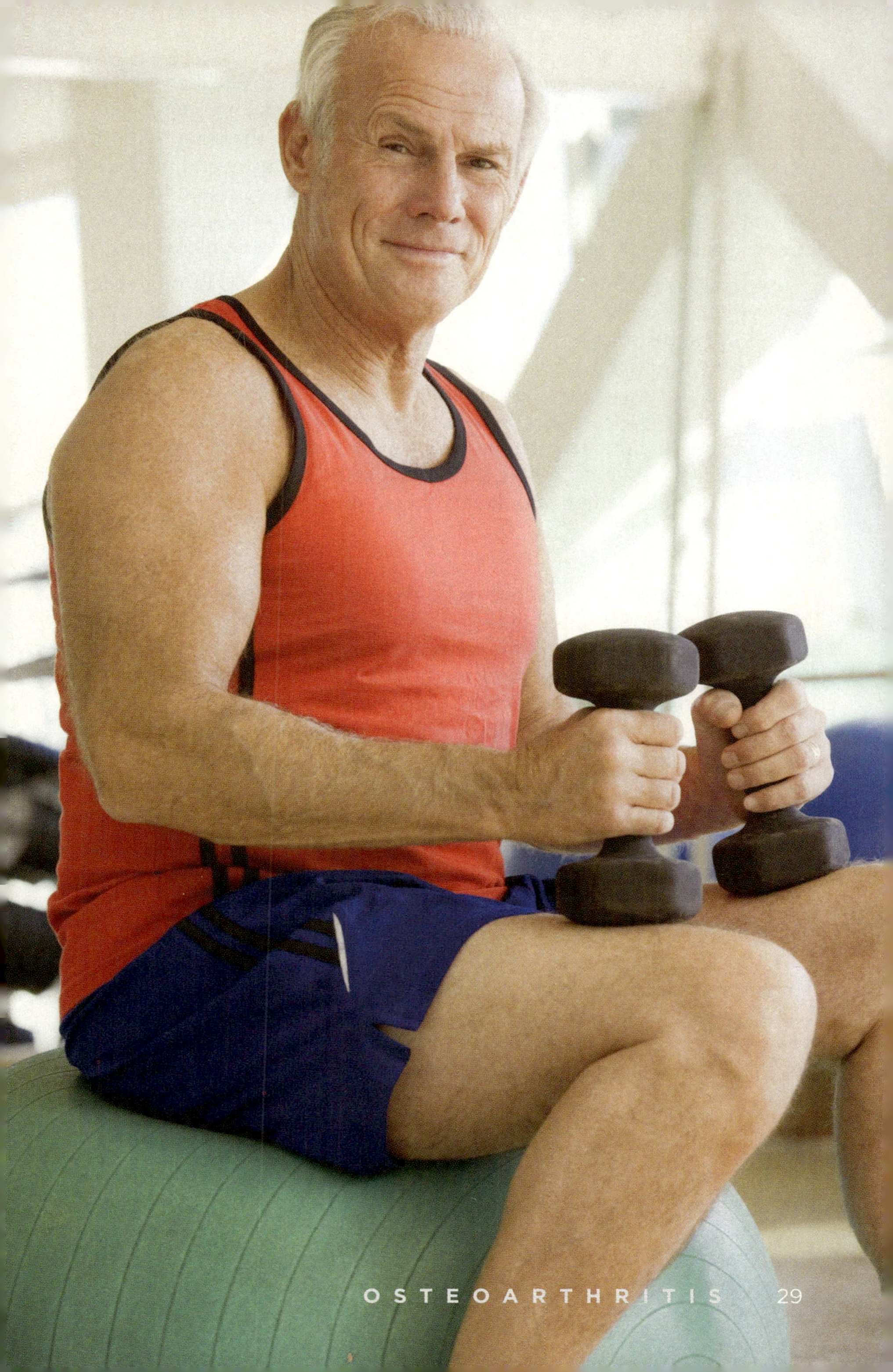

the joint can be corrected with foot orthotics (corrective shoe inserts) or tissue manipulative techniques (chiropractic adjustments, naturopathic manipulations, massage, etc.). Proper alignment of the bones comprising the affected joint, as well as the bones of joints above and below, will relieve pressure on the osteoarthritic joint, lessening pain and improving mobility. These corrections are especially important during exercise so as not to aggravate the effects of joint misalignment on a damaged joint.

Other ways to support the dynamic integrity of joints is through gentle movements. Tai chi and yoga are two types of exercise which encourage flexibility and strength of joints without straining them. These traditions have been developed over centuries and are practiced around the world by people of all ages. Classes and home videos make these activities widely accessible. If these exercises cause discomfort, one may consider receiving acupuncture treatments. Acupuncture can be a great alternative to aspirin for reducing pain and muscle aches, and could be an excellent complement to herbal, exercise and dietary therapies.

Final Thoughts

Osteoarthritis does not have to be the bane of adulthood. We do not have to lose our flexibility, agility and comfort as we age. While the immediate pain relief provided by conventional anti-inflammatory medications may seem appealing, these methods fall far short of actually treating osteoarthritis. Using NSAIDs or aspirin until the point at which surgery becomes the only option is not the only choice for osteoarthritis sufferers. Natural therapies offer a plethora of options. Riding upon the shoulders of glucosamine are newly available, highly concentrated herbal extracts. Boswellia, turmeric, Devil's claw and Indian gooseberry combine powerful anti-inflammatory and antioxidant actions which protect cartilage, reduce pain and support joint stability and flexibility. Using a supplement that contains all four ingredients at the correct concentrations provides a synergistic effect and ensures proper potency.

Supporting the benefits of these herbs is a whole foods diet. This diet provides essential nutrients, minimizes inflammation and helps to eliminate excess weight. Proper exercise completes a holistic healthy joint treatment plan. A comprehensive natural treatment program offers the promise of an active and comfortable life for people with osteoarthritis.

Selected References

Alschuler L and Gazella K. *Definitive Guide to Cancer: An Integrative Approach to Prevention, Treatment, and Healing*. Celestial Arts, 2007.

Antony B, Merina B, Iyer S. et al. A Pilot Cross-over Study to Evaluate Human Oral Bioavailability of BCM-95 CG (Biocurcumax), A Novel Bioenhanced Preparation of Curcumin. *Indian Journal of Pharmaceutical Sciences*. 70:445-450, 2008.

Bland JH, Cooper SM. Osteoarthritis: a review of the cell biology involved and evidence for reversibility. Management rationally related to known genesis and pathophysiology. Seminars in Arthritis and Rheumatism. 14:106-133, 1984.

Childers NF, Margoles MS. An apparent relation of nightshades (Solanaceae) to arthritis. *Journal of Neurological and Orthopaedic Medicine and Surgery*. 14:227–31, 1993.

Deodhar SD, Sethi R, Srimal RC: Preliminary study on antirheumatic activity of curcumin (diferuloyl methane). *Indian Journal of Medical Research* 71:632-634, 1980.

Farrar E, Mitchell H. Osteoarthritis and exercise: a review of the literature. *JSC Medical Association*. 105:8-11, 2009.

Ganju L, Karan D, Chanda S, et al. Immunomodulatory effects of agents of plant origin. *Biomedicine & Pharmacotherapy*. 57:296-300, 2003.

Grazio S, Baleu D. Obesity: risk factor and predictor of osteoarthritis. *Lijec Vjesn*. 131:22-26, 2009.

Kulkarni RR, Patki PS, Jog VP, et al. Treatment of osteoarthritis with a herbomineral formulation: a double-blind, placebo-controlled, cross-over study. Journal of Ethnopharmacology. 33:91-95, 1991.

Lao C, Ruffin M, Normolle D, et al. Dose escalation of a curcuminoid formulation. BMC Complementary and Alternative Medicine. 6:10, 2006.

Lawrence RC, Helmick CG, Arnett FC, et al. Estimates of the prevalence of arthritis and selected musculoskeletal disorders in the United States. *Arthritis and Rheumatism*. 43:778-799, 1998.

Murray M., Pizzorno P., Pizzorno L. *The Encyclopedia of Healing Foods*. Atria Books, 2005.

Noack W, et al. Glucosamine sulfate in osteoarthritis of the knee. *Osteoarthritis Cartilage*. 2:51-59, 1994.

Pizzorno J. and Murray M. *Textbook of Natural Medicine*, 2nd edition. Churchill Livingstone, 1999.

Satoskar RR, Shah SJ, Shenoy SG: Evaluation of anti-inflammatory property of curcumin (diferuloyl methane) in patients with postoperative inflammation. *International Journal of Clinical Pharmacology, Therapy and Toxicology.* 24:651-654, 1986.

Sumantran V, Kulkarni A, Chandwaskar R, et al. Chondroprotective Potential of Fruit Extracts of Phyllanthus emblica in Osteoarthritis. *Evidence-Based Complementary and Alternative Medicine.* 5:329-35, 2008.

Warnock K, McBean D, Suter A, et al. Effectiveness and safety of devil's claw tablets in patients with general rheumatic disorders. *Phytotherapy Research.* 21:1228-1233, 2007.

Wegener T, Lupke N. Treatment of patients with Arthrosis of hip or knee with an aqueous extract of Devil's claw (Harpagophytum procumbens DC). *Phytotherapy Research.* 17:1165-72, 2003.

For more information about the herbs mentioned in this booklet, visit

www.EuroPharmaUSA.com.

For more information about the author of this booklet, visit

www.drlise.net.

CHECK OUT ANOTHER BETTER NUTRITION HEALTHY LIVING GUIDE TODAY!

This booklet is a part of the Better Nutrition Healthy Living Guide *series. For more information about other topics in this series, visit your local independent health food store or visit us online.*

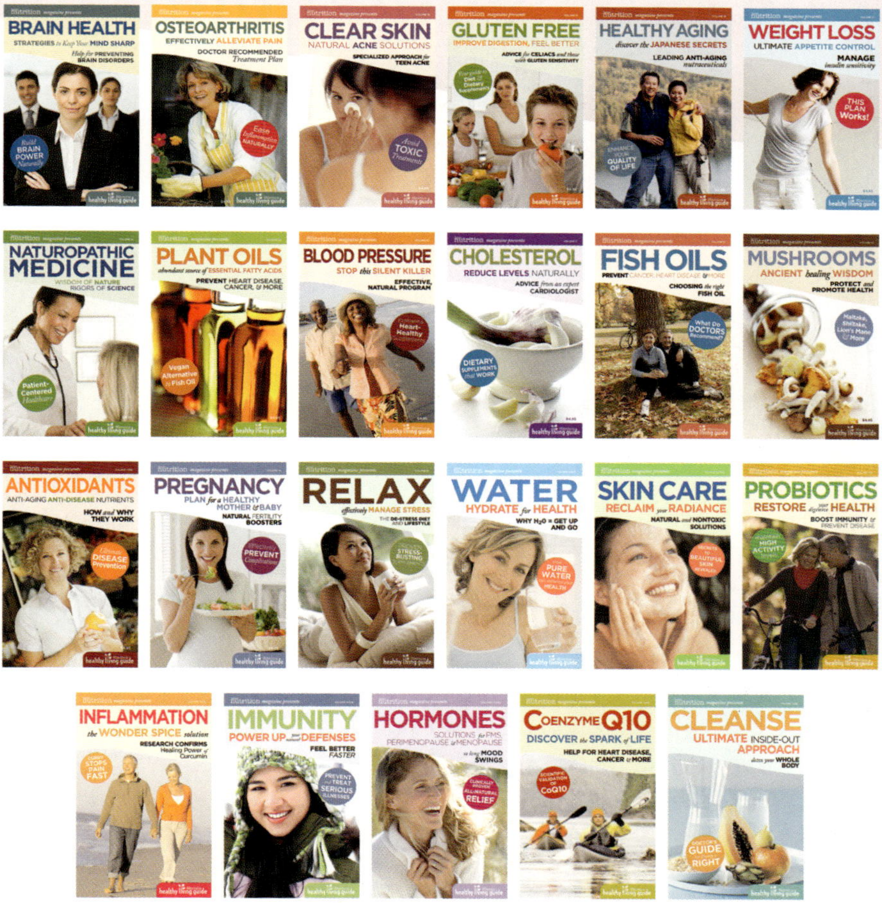

better nutrition healthy living guide

betternutrition.com

better nutrition *magazine presents*

OSTEOARTHRITIS

PROTECT *and* HEAL STIFF AND PAINFUL JOINTS

Osteoarthritis is a painful condition that can become highly debilitating. It is one of the most frequent causes of disability among adults in the United States. Naturopathic clinician and author Lise Alschuler, ND, explains how conventional medicines only address symptoms of osteoarthritis but do not speak to issues of cartilage preservation and repair. In this educational booklet, Dr. Alschuler outlines her plan to help individuals prevent and even reverse osteoarthritis. In addition to directly impacting joint health, her approach also outlines ways to ease pain and inflammation. Before you reach for the aspirin for your joint and back pain, read this booklet.

ABOUT THE AUTHOR OF THIS BOOKLET

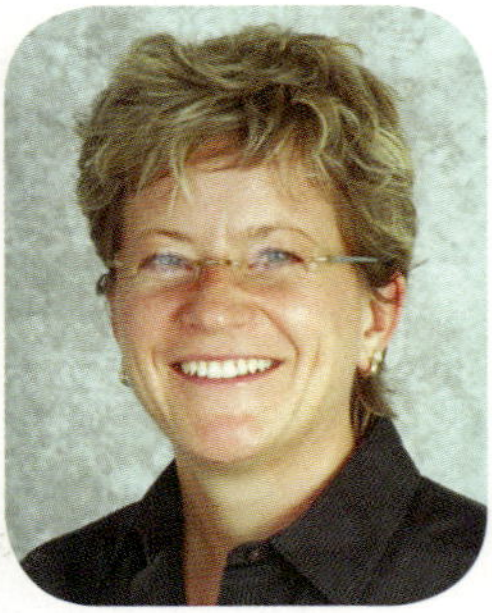

Lise Alschuler, ND, is a naturopathic physician with board certification in naturopathic oncology. She practices naturopathic oncology at Naturopathic Specialists, LLC, in Scottsdale, Ariz. Dr. Alschuler has authored many articles in professional and popular press publications and is the coauthor of the *Definitive Guide to Cancer: An Integrative Approach to Prevention, Treatment and Healing*. She currently serves as president of the American Association of Naturopathic Physicians.

ISBN 978-1-935297-24-6

50495

9 781935 297246

better nutrition healthy living guide

betternutrition.com